ATOMIC TRUST:
A Journey of Trust and Betrayal.

Matthew L. Copeland.

Dedication.

I dedicate this book to God for His matchless and enabling grace. Dedicated to our family—the people who dwell in our hearts and are the unwavering pillars of love and trust. They continue to be our steadfast support system through the highs and lows, helping us navigate the fine line between betrayal and trust. I hope that this voyage across the pages of "Atomic Trust" serves as a reminder of the complex web of relationships and the lasting strength of family ties.

Table of contents

Introduction.

In "Atomic Trust: A Journey of Trust and Betrayal," we examine the fine line that separates trust from betrayal as we dig into the complex dynamics of family and relationships. This novel takes readers on an engrossing trip against the backdrop of contemporary society, one in which loyalty is called into question, friendships are put to the test, and secrets threaten to tear apart the foundation of familial trust. We explore the intricacies of interpersonal relationships via an engrossing story, illuminating the enormous influence of trust and the terrible fallout from Betrayal in the close-knit family. Come along with us as we begin on a moving journey across the turbulent landscape of family ties as we explore love, loyalty, and the enduring endurance of the human spirit.

Chapter 1. Foundations of Trust.

Trust is the foundation of any solid relationship, particularly within the multifaceted elements of family bonds. Inside the setting of family, trust fills in as the bedrock whereupon love, security, and closeness are constructed. Notwithstanding, this trust can be delicate and vulnerable to breaks and disloyalties that can resound through the ages. In this book, we dive into the idea of "atomic Trust" inside family connections, investigating its establishments, appearances, and the significant effects of disloyalty. The Beginning of Confidence in Family: Trust in family connections starts to form from the earliest stages, established by the steady consideration and responsiveness of essential guardians. Children figure out how to trust when their necessities are met quickly and affectionately, encouraging a feeling of safety and connection. As kids develop, trust extends through reliable support, open communication, and common regard within the atomic family. These early encounters shape the groundwork of trust, affecting how people see and explore connections all through their lives.

Atomic Trust, a term instituted by clinician Dr. Kenneth Kaye, alludes to the principal trust people have in their relatives. It envelops the conviction that relatives will act for one another's well being, maintain shared esteem, and offer profound help through various challenges. This trust is seen as atomic, shaping the core of familial bonds and characterizing the substance of relational peculiarities. Be that as it may, the Journey of atomic Trust isn't without its preliminaries. Betrayals inside family connections can break this trust, sending shockwaves through the actual texture of familial associations. Whether through disloyalty, misdirection, or relinquishment, treacheries leave permanent scars, dissolving the groundwork of trust and leaving people wrestling with sensations of Betrayal, outrage, and frustration.

The Ripple Effects of Betrayal:

Treacheries inside family connections have broad results, reaching out past the people directly involved. Kids, specifically, are profoundly impacted by familial treacheries as they battle to accommodate their romanticized view of family with the unforgiving real factors of Betrayal. Seeing parental disagreement or encountering parental betrayal can prompt close-to-home pain and weakness, and trust gives that perseverance into adulthood. Besides, familial treacheries can break the whole family framework, making cracks that partition kin, guardians, and broadened family members. Trust becomes delicate, communication separates, and connections become stressed as relatives wrestle with sensations of harm, hatred, and Betrayal. The once-atomic trust disperses, abandoning a divided scene of broken connections and unsettled clashes.

Rebuilding Trust:
While the effect of Betrayal inside family connections is significant, the Journey towards recuperating isn't difficult to revamp trust. It

requires receptiveness, modesty, and an eagerness to face awkward bits of insight. communication becomes fundamental as relatives participate in fair exchanges, communicating their sentiments and looking for understanding. Pardoning, however, is an urgent step towards modifying trust. It includes relinquishing hatred and outrage, recognizing the humanity of the individuals who have double-crossed us, and embracing sympathy and empathy.

Through pardoning, people can release the hold of past Betrayals, making ready for compromise and recharged associations within the family. Developing Solid Relational Intricacies: Forestalling disloyalties inside family connections starts with developing sound relational peculiarities grounded in straightforwardness, regard, and compassion. Open communication channels cultivate trust, permitting relatives to communicate their requirements, concerns, and limits straightforwardly. Regard for individual independence and office guarantees that every relative feels esteemed and engaged inside the familial unit. Additionally, developing sympathy and understanding inside the family supports the capacity to appreciate anyone on a profound level and cultivates further associations. Sympathy empowers relatives to adjust to one another's feelings, offering help and approval in the midst of euphoria and distress. By developing a culture of compassion, families can sustain the underpinnings of trust, making strong bonds that endure everyday hardships.

All in all, trust is the backbone of family connections, filling in as the paste that ties people together with enamored security and common regard. Atomic Trust, established in the conviction that relatives will act for one another's well being, shapes the core of familial bonds, characterizing the quintessence of relational peculiarities. Nonetheless, treacheries inside family connections can crack this trust, sending shockwaves through the actual texture of familial associations. In spite of the significant effects of betrayal, it is a journey towards mending, and it isn't difficult to revamp trust. Through open communication, absolution, and compassion, families can explore the intricacies of trust, manufacturing more grounded associations and developing tough bonds that get through the everyday hardships.

Chapter 2. Atomic Trust's Inception.

In the domain of human communication, hardly any ideas convey as much weight as trust. It is the establishment whereupon connections are constructed, and its delicacy can disentangle even the most grounded bonds. Inside the complicated embroidery of relational peculiarities, trust assumes a critical role in forming the course of people's lives. "Atomic Trust: A Journey of Trust and Disloyalty" digs into this perplexing exchange, offering a convincing story that investigates the beginning of trust and its resulting Betrayal inside familial connections. The Initiation of Trust: Trust, similar to a fragile seed, is established in the ripe soil of shared encounters, common regard, and steadfast help. In the beginning phases of familial connections, trust frequently blooms easily, supported by the genuine love and mind that describe familial bonds. From the primary hug of a parent to the giggling divided among kin, these minutes laid the foundation for a long period of trust and friendship. In "Atomic Trust," the hero's process starts with the ideal setting of a caring family, where trust streams openly like a delicate stream. Through sincere discussions and shared desires, the relatives form a strong bond based on trust and common comprehension. This underlying phase of trust fills in as the bedrock whereupon the account unfurls, making way for the resulting difficulties and disloyalties that lie ahead. The Delicacy of Trust: In spite of its apparently indestructible nature, trust is a delicate product, vulnerable to the destructive powers of duplicity and Betrayal. In "Atomic Trust," the hero's process takes a turbulent turn as they experience unanticipated hindrances that put their trust under a magnifying glass. From murmured insider facts to stowed-away plans, the family's once-strong groundwork starts to disintegrate under the heaviness of duplicity and question. As the story unfurls, the hero wrestles with the difficult acknowledgment that trust, once broken, isn't effortlessly fixed. Every Betrayal fills in as an unmistakable sign of the weakness innate in human connections, featuring the sensitive harmony among trust and Betrayal inside the familial structure. Through strong narration, "Atomic Trust" explores this unpredictable landscape, investigating the significant effect of disloyalty on the texture of relational peculiarities.

The Life Systems of Betrayal:
Disloyalty, similar to a quiet professional killer, prowls in the shadows, holding back to strike unexpectedly. In "Atomic Trust," Betrayal takes on different structures, going from altogether double dealing to unobtrusive control. As the hero defies the brutal real factors of disloyalty inside their family, they are compelled to go up against their weaknesses and uncertainties, wrestling with the staggering consequences of broken trust. Through nuanced character advancement and multifaceted unexpected developments, "Atomic Trust" unwinds the mind-boggling trap of Betrayal that takes steps to destroy the family. Every disloyalty catalyzes contemplation, provoking the hero to scrutinize

their own convictions and values, notwithstanding affliction. From the tragic disclosure of a long-held mystery to the severe Betrayal of a believed compatriot, the story digs profoundly into the complexities of human instinct, investigating the inspirations driving disloyalty and its enduring results.

The Way to Reclamation:
In the midst of the unrest of Betrayal, "Atomic Trust" offers a good omen as the hero leaves on a journey of recovery and compromise. Through demonstrations of pardoning and understanding, the relatives start to recuperate the injuries of disloyalty, gradually reconstructing the trust that was once lost. As they explore the rough landscape of absolution, the hero comes to understand the genuine force of confidence in encouraging flexibility and strength inside familial connections. In the strong finish of "Atomic Trust," the hero rises out of the pot of disloyalty, changed by the groundbreaking force of trust and pardoning. Through their Journey, they find that while Betrayal might test the

restrictions of trust, it is eventually believed that it wins, manufacturing bonds that are more grounded and stronger than at any other time.

Chapter 3. Establishing Cooperation and Alliances to Build Trust.

Perhaps the most fundamental thread in the complex tapestry of human relationships is still trust. Whether inside the setting of families, kinships, or bigger cultural systems, trust frames the bedrock whereupon significant associations are fabricated. In any case, laying out and sustaining trust can be a complicated Journey, laden with difficulties and valuable open doors for development. In the domain of relational peculiarities, trust takes on significant importance, molding the bonds that integrate people and impacting the course of their collaborations. Inside this unique situation, the idea of "Atomic Trust" arises as a convincing structure through which to investigate the elements of trust and disloyalty inside family connections. Similar to molecules structure the essential units of issue, trust fills in as the basic component whereupon familial bonds are built. Inside the system of Atomic Trust, people depend on a common perspective of shared regard, unwavering quality, and genuineness to explore the intricacies of relational peculiarities. Be that as it may, this Journey isn't without its entanglements, as trust can be delicate and vulnerable to Betrayal.

With regards to family connections, Betrayal can take many structures, going from breaks of certainty to inside and out duplicity. These treacheries can dissolve the trust that frames the groundwork of familial bonds, prompting cracks inside the nuclear family. The Journey of trust and Betrayal inside families is frequently set apart by snapshots of weakness and strength, as people explore the intricate territory of absolution, compromise, and modifying trust.

Laying out Participation and Coalitions
Against the backdrop of Atomic Trust, laying out participation and unions arises as an essential procedure for building and keeping up with trust inside family connections. Participation includes

the readiness of relatives to cooperate towards shared objectives, cultivating a feeling of solidarity and common help. In light of shared values and targets, relatives can fortify their bonds and develop a culture of trust inside the nuclear family. One of the vital parts of laying out participation and coalitions inside families is successful communication. Transparent communication fills in as the foundation of trust, permitting relatives to communicate their necessities, concerns, and assumptions in a valuable way. By encouraging a culture of straightforwardness and responsibility, families can establish a steady climate where trust can thrive.

One more significant part of building collaboration and coalitions inside families is developing compassion and understanding. Compassion includes the capacity to perceive and approve the feelings and points of view of others, encouraging a feeling of association and fortitude. By rehearsing compassion, relatives can construct scaffolds of trust and fortify their connections, even despite difficulties and clashes.

Building Trust Through Cooperation:
Cooperation assumes a fundamental part in building trust inside family connections, as it includes cooperating towards shared objectives and shared goals. By working together on undertakings and tasks, relatives can foster a feeling of collaboration and common regard, laying the preparation for trust to flourish. Cooperation additionally permits relatives to use each other's assets and abilities, setting out open doors for development and advancement. By recognizing and valuing each other's commitments, relatives can develop a culture of regard and profound respect, fortifying their obligations of confidence all the while. Besides, cooperation encourages a feeling of responsibility and interest in the nuclear family, as people feel esteemed and remembered for dynamic cycles. By including relatives in significant conversations and exercises, families can engage every part to take responsibility for

jobs and obligations, encouraging a deep satisfaction and having a place.

End:

In the Journey of Atomic Trust inside family connections, laying out collaboration and partnerships arises as an imperative procedure for building and keeping up with trust. By encouraging powerful communication, compassion, and joint effort, families can develop a culture of trust and versatility, exploring the intricacies of trust and Betrayal with elegance and understanding. As families cooperate towards shared objectives and shared desires, they lay the foundation for persevering through obligations of trust that endure everyday hardship.

Chapter 4. The Betrayal Starts: Indications of Deceit.

At the point when trust is broken, the fallout can be devastating, prompting a Journey of disloyalty and double dealing. In this book, we dive into the complexities of Betrayal inside the setting of family and connections, utilizing the structure of "Atomic Trust" to figure out the elements at play. At the point when this trust is compromised, it can have expansive outcomes, influencing the people directly involved as well as the whole of the relationship or family.

Signs of misleading:

Absence of Straightforwardness: One of the earliest signs of trickery inside a family or relationship is an absence of straightforwardness. At the point when people start to keep data or are shifty about their activities, it can flag hidden issues of doubt.

Irregularities in Conduct:
One more warning is irregularities in conduct. At the point when somebody's activities don't line up with their words or past way of behaving, it can demonstrate underhanded expectations.

Mystery and Secret Plans:
Staying quiet or holding onto stowed-away plans is an obvious sign of being misleading. Whether it's monetary mysteries inside a family or secret thought processes in a relationship, mystery disintegrates trust and establishes the groundwork for Betrayal.

Unexplained Changes in Daily Schedule:
Unexpected changes in everyday practice or unexplained nonappearances can likewise be indications of double dealing. These progressions frequently show a change in needs or the presence of outer impacts that are kept stowed away.

Premonition:
Frequently neglected, however essential, hunches or instincts can make people aware of fundamental double dealing. Focusing on these senses can assist with uncovering stowed-away treacheries before they arise.

In "Atomic Trust," the Journey of trust and Betrayal is a perplexing one, portrayed by different stages:

Foundation of Trust:
At the beginning, there are areas of strength for trust within the family or relationship. People have a good sense of reassurance and are sure about one another's expectations, cultivating a feeling of solidarity and union.

Disloyalty:
The main breaks in trust show up with Betrayal. Whether it's disloyalty, monetary duplicity, or close to home control, the demonstration of Betrayal breaks the "Atomic Trust" and sends

shockwaves through the relationship or nuclear family.

Aftermath and Outcomes:
The result of Betrayal is set apart by the aftermath and outcomes. Trust is broken, and people wrestle with sensations of outrage, Betrayal, and hurt. The elements inside the family or relationship are generally changed, prompting a time of strife and precariousness.

Remaking Trust:
Reconstructing trust is a difficult but fundamental stage in the exploration of "Atomic Trust." It requires open communication, responsibility, and an eagerness to resolve hidden issues. People should show earnestness and consistency in their activities to continuously revamp trust.
Mending and Pushing Ahead:
With time and exertion, recuperating can happen, and people can start to push ahead. While the scars of Betrayal may wait, the experience can at last fortify the bonds inside the

family or relationship, prompting a more profound degree of trust and understanding.

End:
Betrayal inside the setting of family and connections is an intricate and excruciating experience, described by a Journey of trust and Betrayal. By grasping the signs of trickery and exploring the elements of "Atomic Trust," people can stand up to Betrayal, remake trust, and at last arise more grounded from the experience. It is through open communication, sympathy, and a promise to trustworthiness that families and connections can conquer the difficulties of Betrayal and manufacture a way towards recuperating and compromising.

Chapter 5. Rebuilding Trust: Atonement or Retaliation?

In the complicated woven artwork of human connections, trust is the delicate string that keepIns families intact. Be that as it may, when trust is broken, the most common way of modifying it turns into a fragile dance among reparation and reprisal. This Journey of trust and Betrayal, frequently compared to an "Atomic Trust," can leave enduring scars on relational intricacies, testing the actual texture of association and love.

The Groundwork of Trust

Trust inside a family is similar to a holy settlement, worked over long stretches of shared encounters, common regard, and genuine help. It is the foundation whereupon connections flourish, encouraging a conviction that all is good and having a place. However, this establishment can be effectively cracked by activities or words that double-cross the understood comprehension of unwaveringly and genuineness.

The Disloyalty:
A Crack in Atomic Trust
At the point when disloyalty happens inside the nuclear family, it sends shockwaves through the actual center of connections, upsetting the fragile equilibrium of trust. Whether it's unfaithfulness, trickery, or break of certainty, the aftermath from such activities can be devastating, leaving close to home injuries that run profound.

"Atomic Trust," as it is frequently alluded to, depicts the dangerous idea of Betrayal inside familial bonds. Very much like an atomic response, the results of broken trust can be sweeping, influencing the people straightforwardly involved as well as undulating out to affect the whole relational intricacy.

Exploring the fallout of Betrayal requires a fragile dance among compensation and counter. For the deceived, the way to recuperating is laden with vulnerability and inner unrest. Inquiries of pardoning, recovery, and the chance of reconstructing trust pose a potential threat, creating a shaded area over the once-strong groundwork of family bonds.

Then again, the deceiver should stand up to their activities, wrestling with sensations of culpability, regret, and the results of their Betrayal. The Journey of reparation is laden with its own difficulties, requiring certified contemplation, responsibility, and a readiness to set things straight.

Penance:
The Way to Reconstructing Trust. For some purposes, penance turns into an encouraging sign in the midst of the obscurity of Betrayal. It is a Journey of self-disclosure and reclamation, portrayed by genuine statements of regret, sincere regret, and substantial endeavors to right the wrongs committed. Through demonstrations of lowliness and certified regret, the deceiver

looks to acquire back the trust that was lost, crawling towards compromise and mending.

Penance is certainly not a clear way, in any case. It requires persistence, modesty, and a readiness to face awkward insights. It includes dealing with the outcomes of one's activities directly, setting things straight, and exhibiting a veritable obligation to change. Just through steady exertion and authentic regret could the double-crosser at any point desire to modify the broken trust and retouch the break in Atomic Trust.

Reprisal:
The Allurement of Retaliation
However, in the midst of the unrest of Betrayal, the enticement of reprisal poses a potential threat. Reprisal, driven by sensations of outrage, disdain, and a longing for equity, can appear in different structures - from profound withdrawal and latent forceful way of behaving to through and through conflict and looking for retribution.

While reprisal might offer a passing feeling of fulfillment, it at last propagates a pattern of harm and questioning, further developing the injuries brought about by Betrayal. Rather than cultivating mending and compromise, it just draws out the torment and sustains a pattern of harmfulness inside the nuclear family.

The Way ahead:
Recuperating and Compromise
Right after Betrayal, the way ahead is loaded with difficulties, yet it likewise holds the commitment of mending and compromise. It requires an aggregate obligation to confront the excruciating insights, take part in transparent communication, and develop a culture of sympathy, pardoning, and unrestricted love.

Revamping trust inside the family is a journey that requires persistence, constancy, and an eagerness to embrace weakness. It includes recognizing the aggravation brought about by Betrayal, yet additionally clutching the expectation of recovery and recharging. Through demonstrations of certified regret, genuine conciliatory sentiments, and a promise to change, the deceiver can start to procure back the trust that was lost, laying the preparation for recuperating and compromise.

End:

In the complicated scene of family connections, trust is the delicate string that ties hearts together. At the point when trust is broken by disloyalty, the Journey of reconstructing it turns into a fragile dance among penance and reprisal. However, in the midst of the aggravation and unrest, there is likewise the chance of mending and compromise. Through demonstrations of certified regret, earnest expressions of remorse, and a promise to change, families can explore the wild waters of disloyalty and arise more grounded, stronger, and bound together by a recently discovered feeling of trust and love.

Chapter 6. Lessons Acquired: The Consequences of Betrayal.

Atomic Trust: A Journey of Trust and Betrayal" digs into the intricacies of familial connections, investigating the complex transaction among trust and Betrayal and the enduring illustrations obtained from these encounters.

Disloyalty inside the nuclear family can take many structures, going from Betrayal and duplicity to relinquishment and disregard. No matter what its appearance, disloyalty makes a permanent imprint on both the deceiver and the sold out, reshaping their discernments and adjusting the direction of their connections. "Atomic Trust" enlightens this extraordinary cycle, showing how Betrayal can break the deception of safety and uncover the weaknesses innate in familial associations.

One of the most significant illustrations gathered from "Atomic Trust" is the acknowledgment that trust is a sensitive equilibrium, effortlessly disturbed by the activities of those nearest to us. The hero's process features the intrinsic dangers related with setting steady confidence in others, highlighting the significance of wisdom and self-conservation. Through the turbulent exciting bends in the road of their familial adventure, they come to comprehend that trust should be procured through predictable activities and authentic earnestness, as opposed to dazed faithfulness.

Besides, "Atomic Trust" highlights the intricacies of absolution in the consequence of Betrayal. While pardoning is much of the time proclaimed as a way to recuperate and compromise, it is a profoundly private and nuanced process that can't be surged or constrained. The hero wrestles with clashing feelings as they explore the wild waters of pardoning, grappling with sensations of outrage, hatred, and at last, acknowledgment. Their process fills in as a strong update that pardoning isn't inseparable from neglecting or supporting the activities of the traitor yet rather a method for setting oneself free from the shackles of sharpness and hatred.

Additionally, "Atomic Trust" reveals insight into the expanding influences of Betrayal inside the familial biological system, penetrating resulting ages and molding their impression of trust and closeness. The hero's kids are not insusceptible to the scars left by their folks' treacheries, wrestling with their own uncertainties and separation anxieties. Through their battles, "Atomic Trust" highlights the intergenerational transmission of trust issues, accentuating the requirement for open communication and weakness to break the pattern of Betrayal.

Eventually, "Atomic Trust" fills in as a piercing investigation of the delicacy of trust and the persevering through versatility of the human soul despite Betrayal. It advises us that while disloyalty might crack familial bonds, it additionally presents a chance for development, self-revelation, and eventually, reclamation. By standing up to the outcomes of Betrayal head-on, the hero arises more grounded, smarter, and more sensitive to the complexities of trust and closeness.

All in all, "Atomic Trust: A Journey of Trust and Betrayal" offers priceless bits of knowledge into the outcomes of Betrayal inside the familial setting, featuring the extraordinary force of pardoning, versatility, and self-disclosure. Through the hero's Journey, we are helped to remember the persevering through significance of confidence in supporting solid, satisfying connections and the significant illustrations obtained through the cauldron of disloyalty. As we explore the intricacies of familial elements, may we stay cautious gatekeepers of trust, perceiving its innate delicacy and appreciating its significant ability to enhance our lives.

Conclusion.

Through the characters' trials and triumphs, we have seen the enduring power of empathy, forgiveness, and communication in navigating the complexities of human connections. As the journey comes to an end, it is clear that while trust is brittle and easily broken, it is also resilient and can be rebuilt with patience, understanding, and a willingness to face the shadows of betrayal. In essence, "Atomic Trust: A Journey of Trust and Betrayal" reminds us that the bonds of family and relationships are both fragile and enduring, shaped by the decisions we make and the courage we exhibit in times of adversity.

Acknowledgement.

My family, whose unfailing love and support have been the cornerstone of my journey in creating this book, has my sincere appreciation. I am grateful to my parents for establishing in me the virtues of perseverance, honesty, and trust that permeate these pages. Thank you to my siblings for their support and tolerance when I worked long hours at my desk.

I am also really grateful to my partner, who has been there for me no matter how much our time together has been taken up by the demands of this project. Your steadfast assistance has served as my compass during the choppy waters of invention. I will always be appreciative of your generosity and thoughtfulness.

Finally, I just wanted to say thank you to all of my readers. Your curiosity for the intricacies of trust and Betrayal in the framework of relationships and families has motivated me to learn more about these subjects.

This book is dedicated to everyone who has ever witnessed the complex dance between trust and betrayal in their own lives, as well as to the continuing strength of forgiveness and love in the face of even the most severe betrayals.

About the Publisher.

Through thought-provoking literature, Erudite Publishing is committed to raising awareness and understanding of family dynamics and relationships. The book "Atomic Trust" delves at the intricate dynamics of trust and treachery within familial bonds. The ultimate goal is to improve readers' lives and assist them in developing stronger relationships with those around them by promoting empathy, comprehension, and communication.